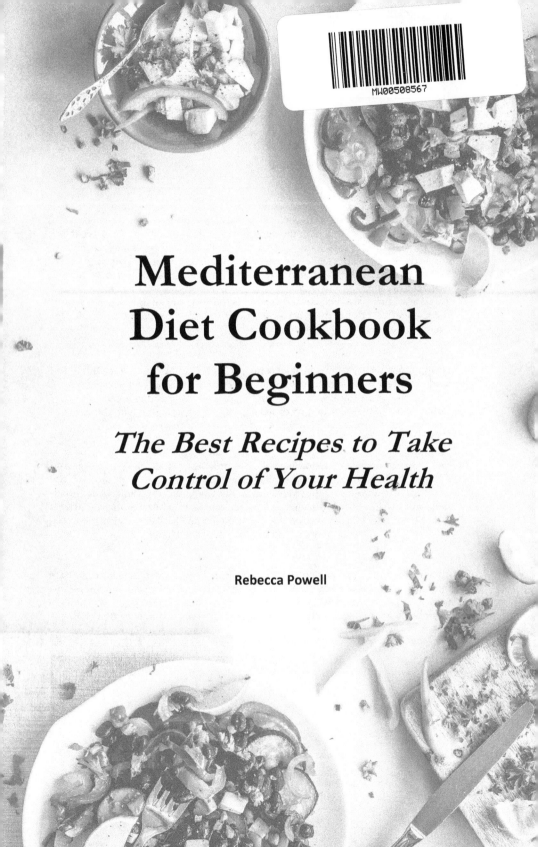

# Mediterranean Diet Cookbook for Beginners

## *The Best Recipes to Take Control of Your Health*

Rebecca Powell

VEGGIES..................................................................5

Traditional Falafel...................................................6

Spicy Split Pea Tabbouleh......................................8

Mashed Avocado Egg Salad with Crisps............11

Healthy Vegetable Medley...................................12

Mediterranean Brussels Sprouts.........................14

Healthy Garlic Eggplant........................................16

Indian Bell Peppers and Potato Stir Fry.............18

Carrot Potato Medley............................................20

Honey Sweet Potatoes:.........................................22

Flavors Basil Lemon Ratatouille..........................23

PASTA RECIPES......................................................25

Sausage Pasta.........................................................26

Pomodoro Pasta.....................................................28

Fra Diavolo Pasta Sauce.......................................32

Ranch Bacon Pasta Salad......................................34

Alfredo Peppered Shrimp.....................................37

Bow Ties with Sausages, Tomatoes & Cream.....39

Penne with Spicy Vodka Tomato Cream Sauce..41

Milanese Chicken...................................................44

One Pan Orecchiette Pasta...................................46

Rustic Pasta............................................................48

Creamy Cajun Chicken Pasta................................51

PIZZA RECIPES.......................................................53

Balsamic-Glazed Pizza with Arugula & Olives....54

Pepperoni Fat Head Pizza.....................................56

Extra Cheesy Pizza.................................................59

Spanish-Style Pizza de Jamon..............................61

Spicy & Smoky Pizza..............................................63

Turkey Pizza with Pesto Topping........................65

Baby Spinach Pizza with Sweet Onion................67

Italian Mushroom Pizza........................................69

Broccoli-Pepper Pizza ...................................................72

White Pizza with Prosciutto and Arugula ..........................74

Za'atar Pizza ...............................................................75

Broccoli Cheese Burst Pizza ...........................................77

Mozzarella Bean Pizza ..................................................79

Pizza Dough Without Yeast in Milk ..................................80

Ideal Pizza Dough (On A Large Baking Sheet)..................82

Vegetable Oil Pizza Dough .............................................84

Pizza Dough on Yogurt...................................................85

Eggplant Pizza .............................................................86

Mediterranean Whole Wheat Pizza ..................................88

Fruit Pizza...................................................................89

Sprouts Pizza ...............................................................90

Cheese Pinwheels..........................................................91

APPETIZERS AND SNACKS.............................................92

Tomato Olive Salsa........................................................93

Thin-Crust Flatbread .....................................................94

Smoked Salmon Goat Cheese Endive Bites.......................96

Hummus Peppers ..........................................................97

Loaded Mediterranean Hummus.......................................98

Smoky Loaded Eggplant Dip ...........................................99

Peanut Butter Banana Greek Yogurt Bowl ......................101

Roasted Chickpeas.......................................................102

Savory Feta Spinach and Sweet Red Pepper Muffins...104

Baked Whole-Grain Lavash Chips with Dip .....................106

Quinoa Granola............................................................108

# VEGGIES

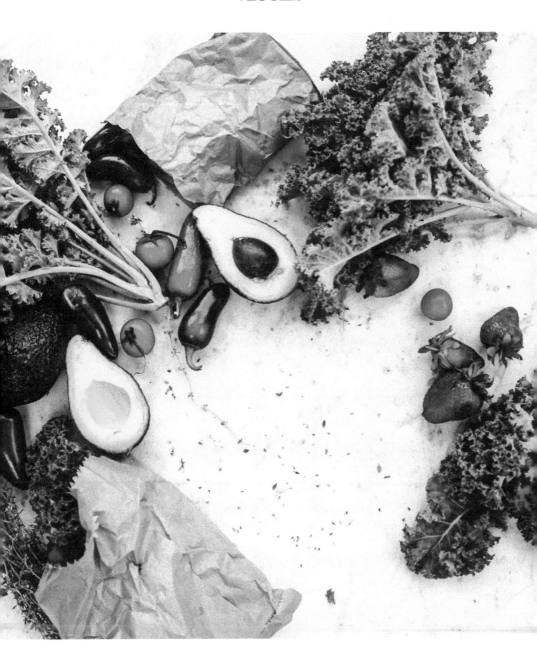

# Traditional Falafel

**Preparation time:** 15 minutes

**Cooking time:** 10 minutes

**Servings:** 4

## INGREDIENTS:

- ☐ 1 (15-ounce) can low-sodium chickpeas, drained and rinsed
- ☐ ½ sweet onion, chopped
- ☐ ¼ cup whole-wheat flour
- ☐ ¼ cup coarsely chopped fresh parsley
- ☐ ¼ cup coarsely chopped fresh cilantro
- ☐ Juice from 1 lemon
- ☐ 1 tablespoon minced garlic
- ☐ 2 teaspoon ground cumin
- ☐ Sea salt
- ☐ Freshly ground black pepper
- ☐ 2 tablespoons olive oil

## INSTRUCTIONS:

**1.** In a food processor, pulse the chickpeas, onion, flour, parsley, cilantro, lemon juice, garlic, and cumin until the mixture just holds together. Season with salt and pepper and mix again.

**2.** Scoop out about 2 tablespoons of the mixture, roll into a ball, and flatten it out slightly to form a thick patty. Repeat with the remaining chickpea mixture.

**3.** In a large skillet, heat the olive oil over medium-high heat and pan-fry the patties until golden brown, about 4 minutes per side. Serve alone or stuffed into pita bread.

**PER SERVING:** Calories: 245 Fat: 9g Carbohydrates: 36g Protein: 7g

# Spicy Split Pea Tabbouleh

**Preparation time:** 15 minutes

**Cooking time:** 45 minutes

**Servings:** 6

## INGREDIENTS:

- ☐ 1½ cups split peas
- ☐ 4 cups water
- ☐ 2 large tomatoes, seeded and chopped
- ☐ 1 English cucumber, chopped
- ☐ 1 yellow bell pepper, chopped
- ☐ 1 orange bell pepper, chopped
- ☐ ½ red onion, finely chopped
- ☐ ¼ cup chopped fresh cilantro
- ☐ Juice of 1 lime
- ☐ 1 teaspoon ground cumin
- ☐ ½ teaspoon ground coriander
- ☐ Pinch red pepper flakes
- ☐ Sea salt
- ☐ Freshly ground black pepper

## INSTRUCTIONS:

**1.** In a large saucepan, combine the split peas and water over medium-high heat and bring to a boil. Reduce the heat to low and simmer, uncovered, until the peas are tender, 40 to 45 minutes. Drain the peas and rinse them in cold water to cool.

**2.** Transfer the peas to a large bowl and add the tomatoes, cucumber, bell peppers, onion, cilantro, lime juice, cumin, coriander, and red pepper flakes. Toss to mix well.

**3.** Place the mixture in the refrigerator for at least 1 hour to let the flavors mesh. Season with salt and pepper and serve.

**PER SERVING:** Calories: 208 Fat: 1g Carbohydrates: 38g Protein: 14g

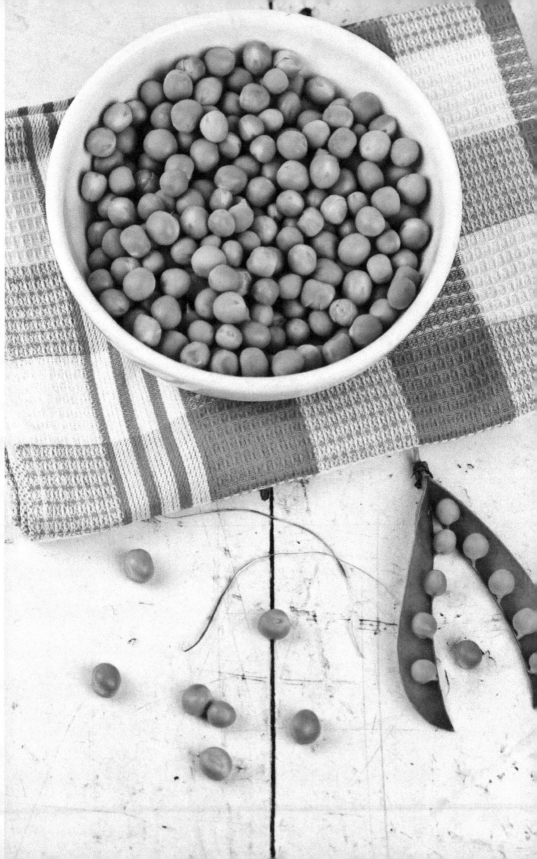

# Mashed Avocado Egg Salad with Crisps

**Preparation time:** 15 minutes

**Cooking time:** 0 minutes

**Servings:** 4

## INGREDIENTS:

- ☐ 6 hard-boiled eggs, peeled and coarsely chopped
- ☐ 1 avocado, peeled and pitted
- ☐ 1 celery stalk, chopped
- ☐ Juice and zest of ½ lemon
- ☐ 1 teaspoon chopped fresh parsley
- ☐ 4 whole-wheat bread slices, toasted
- ☐ 2 tomatoes, thinly sliced
- ☐ Sea salt
- ☐ Freshly ground black pepper

## INSTRUCTIONS:

**1.** In a medium bowl, mash the eggs and avocado until well blended but still chunky. Stir in the celery, lemon juice, lemon zest, and parsley until well mixed.

**2.** Generously spread the egg mixture on the toast and arrange the tomato slices on top. Season with salt and pepper and serve.

**PER SERVING:** Calories: 248 Fat: 14g Carbohydrates: 18g Protein: 13g

# Healthy Vegetable Medley

**Preparation time:** 15 minutes

**Cooking time:** 12 minutes

**Servings:** 6

## INGREDIENTS:

- ☐ 3 cups broccoli florets
- ☐ 1 sweet potato, chopped
- ☐ 1 teaspoon garlic, minced
- ☐ 14 oz. coconut milk
- ☐ 28 oz. can tomato, chopped
- ☐ 14 oz. can chickpeas, drained and rinsed
- ☐ 1 onion, chopped
- ☐ 1 tablespoon olive oil
- ☐ 1 teaspoon Italian seasoning
- ☐ Pepper
- ☐ Salt

## INSTRUCTIONS:

**1.** Add oil into the inner pot of pot and set the pot on sauté

mode. Add garlic and onion and sauté until onion is softened.

**2.** Add remaining ingredients and stir everything well. Seal pot with

lid and cook on high for 12 minutes.

**3.** Once done, allow to release pressure naturally for 10 minutes

then release remaining using quick release. Remove lid.Stir well and serve.

**PER SERVING:** Calories: 322 Fat: 19.3 g Carbs: 34.3 g Protein: 7.9 g

# Mediterranean Brussels Sprouts

**Preparation time:** 15 minutes

**Cooking time:** 23 minutes

**Servings:** 4

## INGREDIENTS:

- ☐ 2 cups Brussels sprouts, cut in half
- ☐ ¼ cup feta cheese, crumbled
- ☐ ¼ cup olive oil
- ☐ 1 bay leaf
- ☐ 2 teaspoons pine nuts, roasted
- ☐ ½ cup olives
- ☐ 2 tablespoons sun-dried tomatoes, chopped
- ☐ Pepper
- ☐ Salt

## INSTRUCTIONS:

**1.** Preheat the oven to 3500 F. Heat 1 tablespoon of oil in a pan over medium heat. Add Brussels sprouts and salt and cook for 7-8 minutes. Place pan in oven and bake sprouts of 10 minutes.

**2.** Meanwhile, in separate pan heat remaining oil over medium heat. Add sun-dried tomatoes and olives and cook for 5 minutes.

**3.** Remove sprouts from oven and mix with tomato olive mixture. Top with crumbled cheese and pine nuts. Serve and enjoy.

**PER SERVING:** Calories: 182 Fat: 17.5 g Carbs: 5.9 g Protein: 3.2 g

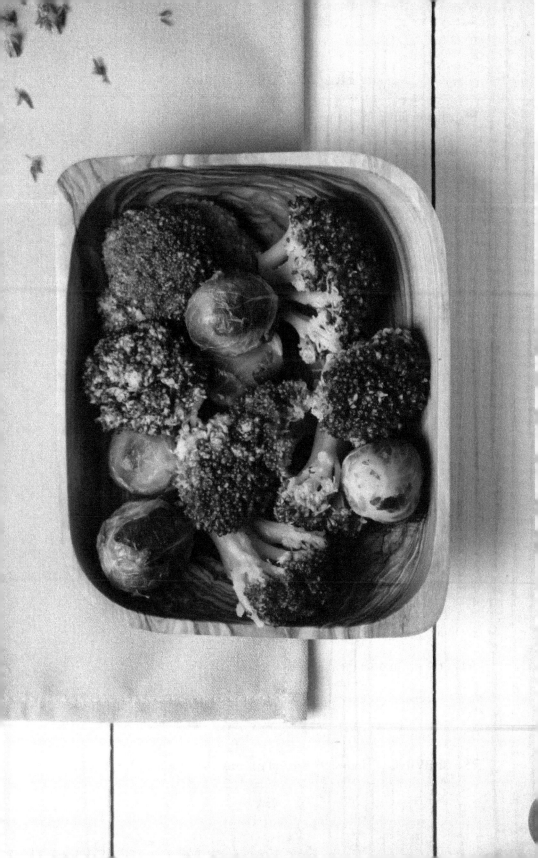

# Healthy Garlic Eggplant

**Preparation time:** 15 minutes

**Cooking time:** 5 minutes

**Servings:** 4

**INGREDIENTS:**

- [ ] 1 eggplant, cut into 1-inch pieces
- [ ] ½ cup of water
- [ ] ¼ cup Can tomato, crushed
- [ ] ½ teaspoon Italian seasoning
- [ ] 1 teaspoon paprika
- [ ] ½ teaspoon chili powder
- [ ] 1 teaspoon garlic powder
- [ ] 2 tablespoons olive oil
- [ ] Salt

**INSTRUCTIONS:**

**1.** Add water and eggplant into the pot. Seal pot with lid and cook on high for 5 minutes. Once done, release pressure using quick release. Remove lid.

**2.** Drain eggplant well and clean the pot. Add oil into the inner pot of the pot and set the pot on sauté mode.

**3.** Add eggplant along with remaining ingredients and stir well and cook for 5 minutes. Serve and enjoy.

**PER SERVING:** Calories: 97 Fat: 7.5 g Carbs: 8.2 g Protein: 1.5 g

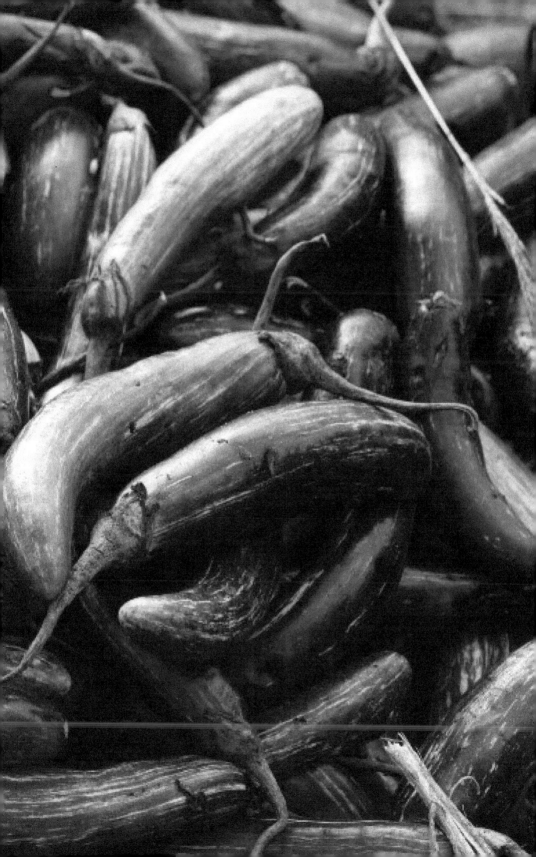

# Indian Bell Peppers and Potato Stir Fry

**Preparation time:** 15 minutes

**Cooking time:** 10 minutes

**Servings:** 2

## INGREDIENTS:

- [ ] 1 tablespoon oil
- [ ] ½ teaspoon cumin seeds
- [ ] 4 cloves of garlic, minced
- [ ] 4 potatoes, scrubbed and halved
- [ ] Salt and pepper to taste
- [ ] 5 tablespoons water
- [ ] 2 bell peppers, seeded and julienned
- [ ] Chopped cilantro for garnish

## INSTRUCTIONS:

**1.** Heat oil in a skillet over medium flame and toast the cumin seeds until fragrant. Add the garlic until fragrant. Stir in the potatoes, salt, pepper, water, and bell peppers.

**2.** Close the lid and allow to simmer for at least 10 minutes. Garnish with cilantro before cooking time ends. Place in individual containers.

**3.** Put a label and store it in the fridge. Allow thawing at room temperature before heating in the microwave oven.

**PER SERVING:** Calories: 83 Fat: 6.4 g Carbs: 7.3 g Protein: 2.8 g

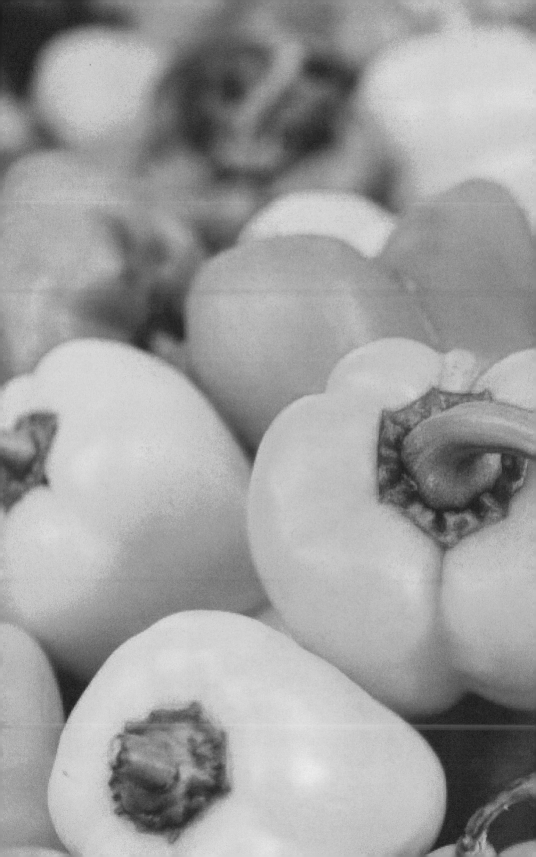

# Carrot Potato Medley

**Preparation time:** 15 minutes

**Cooking time:** 15 minutes

**Servings:** 6

## INGREDIENTS:

- [ ] 4 lbs. baby potatoes, clean and cut in half
- [ ] 1 ½ lb. carrots, cut into chunks
- [ ] 1 teaspoon Italian seasoning
- [ ] 1 ½ cups vegetable broth
- [ ] 1 tablespoon garlic, chopped
- [ ] 1 onion, chopped
- [ ] 2 tablespoons olive oil
- [ ] Pepper
- [ ] Salt

## INSTRUCTIONS:

**1.** Add oil into the inner pot of the pot and set the pot on

sauté mode. Add onion and sauté for 5 minutes. Add carrots and

cook for 5 minutes.

**2.** Add remaining ingredients and stir well. Seal pot with lid and cook

on high for 5 minutes.

**3.** Once done, allow to release pressure naturally for 10 minutes

then release remaining using quick release. Remove lid. Stir and

serve.

**PER SERVING:** Calories: 283 Fat: 5.6 g Carbs: 51.3 g Protein: 10.2 g

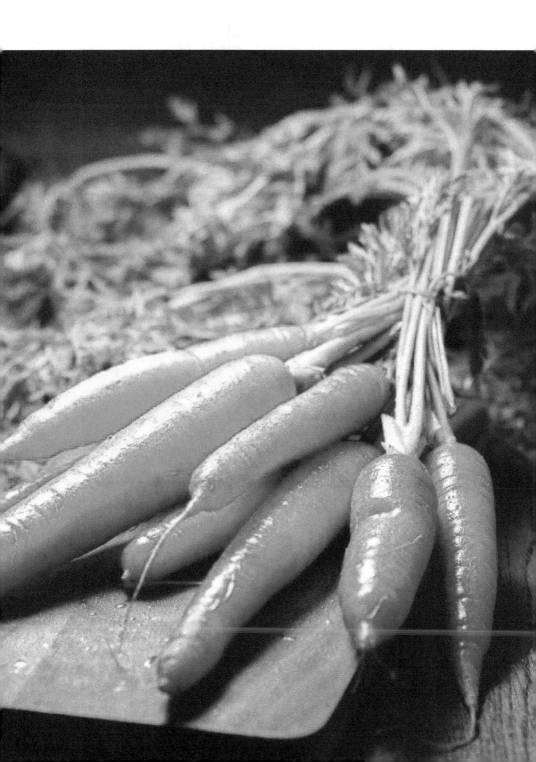

# Honey Sweet Potatoes:

**Preparation time**: 15 minutes

**Cooking time:** 35 minutes

**Servings:** 8

## INGREDIENTS:

- [ ] 4 large sweet potatoes, peel and cut into 1-inch cubes
- [ ] ¼ teaspoon paprika
- [ ] 2 tablespoons olive oil
- [ ] 8 sage leaves
- [ ] 1 teaspoon honey
- [ ] 2 teaspoons vinegar
- [ ] ½ teaspoon of sea salt

## INSTRUCTIONS:

**1.** Preheat the oven to 3750 F. Add sweet potato, olive oil, sage, and salt in a large bowl and toss well.Roast for 35 minutes.

**2.** Add honey, vinegar, and paprika and mix well.Serve and enjoy.

**PER SERVING:** Calories: 90 Fat: 3.5 g Carbs: 14 g Protein: 1 g

# Flavors Basil Lemon Ratatouille

**Preparation time:** 15 minutes

**Cooking time:** 10 minutes

**Servings:** 8

## INGREDIENTS:

- ☐ 1 small eggplant, cut into cubes
- ☐ 1 cup fresh basil
- ☐ 2 cups grape tomatoes
- ☐ 1 onion, chopped
- ☐ 2 summer squash, sliced
- ☐ 2 zucchinis, sliced
- ☐ 2 tablespoons vinegar
- ☐ 2 tablespoons tomato paste
- ☐ 1 tablespoon garlic, minced
- ☐ 1 fresh lemon juice
- ☐ ¼ cup olive oil
- ☐ Salt

## INSTRUCTIONS:

**1.** Add basil, vinegar, tomato paste, garlic, lemon juice, oil, and salt into the blender and blend until smooth. Add eggplant, tomatoes, onion, squash, and zucchini into the pot.

**2.** Pour blended basil mixture over vegetables and stir well. Seal pot with lid and cook on high for 10 minutes. Once done, allow to release pressure naturally. Remove lid. Stir well and serve.

**PER SERVING:** Calories: 103 Fat: 6.8 g Carbs: 10.6 g Protein: 2.4 g

### Roasted Parmesan Cauliflower

**Preparation time:** 15 minutes

**Cooking time:** 30 minutes

**Servings:** 4

## INGREDIENTS:

- ☐ 8 cups cauliflower florets
- ☐ 1 teaspoon dried marjoram
- ☐ 2 tablespoons olive oil
- ☐ ½ cup parmesan cheese, shredded
- ☐ 2 tablespoons vinegar
- ☐ ¼ teaspoon pepper
- ☐ ¼ teaspoon salt

## INSTRUCTIONS:

**1.** Preheat the oven to 4500 F. Toss cauliflower, marjoram, oil, pepper, and salt. Toss well. Spread cauliflower onto the baking tray and roast for 15-20 minutes.

**2.** Toss cauliflower with cheese and vinegar. Return cauliflower to the oven and roast for 5-10 minutes more. Serve and enjoy.

**PER SERVING:** Calories: 196 Fat: 13 g Carbs: 11 g Protein: 11 g

# PASTA RECIPES

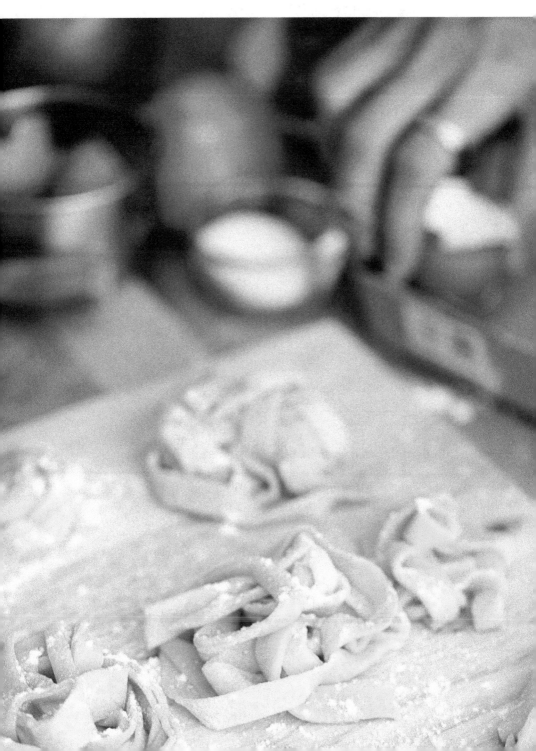

# Sausage Pasta

**Preparation time:** 15 minutes

**Cooking time:** 20 minutes

**Servings:** 6

## INGREDIENTS:

- [ ] 3/4 pound of pasta
- [ ] 1 tablespoon of olive oil
- [ ] Spicy Italian sausage of 1 pound
- [ ] 1 onion, minced
- [ ] 4 cloves of chopped garlic
- [ ] 1 canned chicken broth
- [ ] 1 teaspoon dried basil
- [ ] 1 can diced tomatoes
- [ ] 1 pack (10 oz) of frozen chopped spinach
- [ ] 1/2 cup of grated Parmesan cheese

## INSTRUCTIONS:

**1.** Boil lightly salted water in a large pot, then add pasta and cook until al dente; (8-10 minutes). Drain and set aside.

**2.** Heat oil and sausage in a large skillet; cook until pink. Add the onion and garlic to the pan during the last 5 minutes of cooking. Add the stock, basil, and tomatoes with the liquid.

**3.** Simmer over medium heat for 5 minutes to reduce slightly. Add the chopped spinach; cover the pan and simmer over low heat until the spinach is soft.

**4.** Add the pasta to the pan and mix. Sprinkle with cheese and serve immediately.

**PER SERVING:** Calories 423 Fat 19.3 g Carbohydrates 39 g Protein 22.3 g

# Pomodoro Pasta

**Preparation time:** 15 minutes

**Cooking time:** 25 minutes

**Servings:** 4

## INGREDIENTS:

- ☐ 1 pack of 16 angel hair pasta
- ☐ 1/4 cup of olive oil
- ☐ 1/2 onion, minced
- ☐ 4 cloves of chopped garlic
- ☐ 2 cups of Roma tomatoes, diced
- ☐ 2 tablespoons balsamic vinegar
- ☐ 1 low-sodium chicken broth
- ☐ ground red pepper
- ☐ freshly ground black pepper to taste
- ☐ 1/4 cup grated Parmesan cheese
- ☐ 2 tablespoons chopped fresh basil

## INSTRUCTIONS:

**1.** Bring a large pot of lightly salted water to a boil. Add pasta and cook for 8 minutes or until al dente; drain.

**2.** Pour the olive oil in a large deep pan over high heat. Fry onions and garlic until light brown. Lower the heat to medium and add tomatoes, vinegar, and chicken stock; simmer for about 8 minutes.

**3.** Stir in the red pepper, black pepper, basil, and cooked pasta and mix well with the sauce. Simmer for about 5 minutes and serve garnished with grated cheese.

**PER SERVING:** Calories 500 Fat 18.3 g Carbohydrates 69.7 g Protein 16.2 g

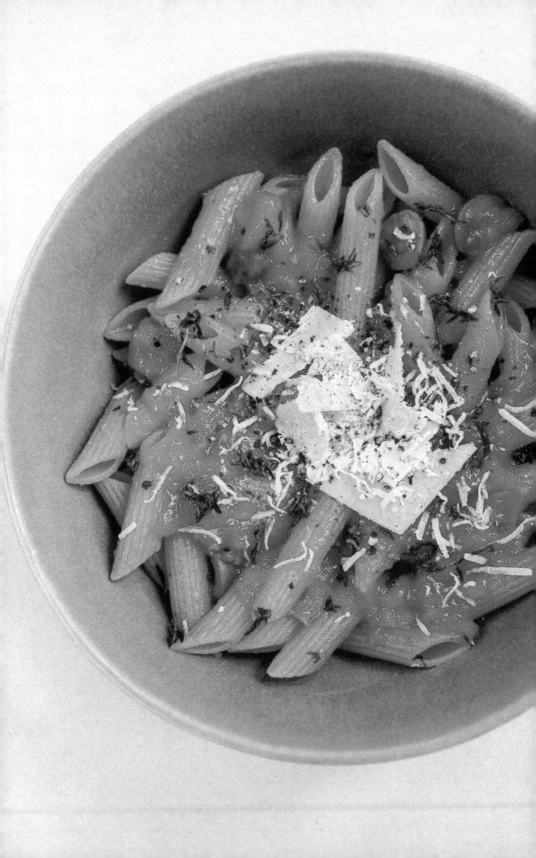

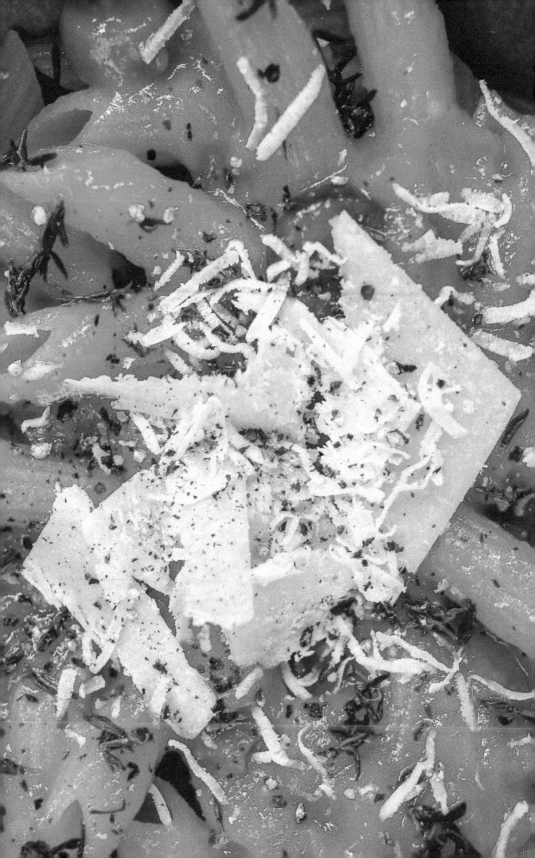

# Fra Diavolo Pasta Sauce

**Preparation time:** 15 minutes

**Cooking time:** 55 minutes

**Servings:** 8

## INGREDIENTS:

- ☐ 4 tablespoons olive oil, divided
- ☐ 6 cloves of garlic, crushed
- ☐ 3 cups peeled whole tomatoes with liquid, chopped
- ☐ 1 1/2 teaspoon of salt
- ☐ 1 teaspoon crushed red pepper flakes
- ☐ 1 packet of linguine pasta
- ☐ 8 grams of small shrimp, peeled
- ☐ 8 grams of bay scallops
- ☐ 1 tablespoon of chopped fresh parsley

## INSTRUCTIONS:

**1.** Heat 2 tablespoons of olive oil and sauté garlic over medium heat.

When the garlic starts to sizzle, pour in the tomatoes.

**2.** Season with salt and red pepper. Bring to boil. Reduce the heat

and simmer for 30 minutes, stirring occasionally.

**3.** Meanwhile, boil a large pan with lightly salted water. Cook pasta

for about 8 to 10 minutes or until al dente; drain.

**4.** Heat the remaining 2 tablespoons of olive oil in a large frying pan

over high heat. Add shrimps and scallops. Cook for about 2

minutes stirring regularly, or until the shrimp turn pink.

**5.** Add the shrimp and scallops to the tomato mixture and stir in the parsley. Bake for 3 to 4 minutes or until the sauce starts to bubble. Serve the sauce on the pasta.

**PER SERVING:** Calories 335 Fat 8.9 g Carbohydrates 46.3 g Protein 18.7 g

# Ranch Bacon Pasta Salad

**Preparation time:** 15 minutes

**Cooking time:** 15 minutes

**Servings:** 10

## INGREDIENTS:

- 1 (12 oz.) package of uncooked tri color rotini
- 10 slices of bacon
- 1 cup mayonnaise
- 3 tablespoons dry ranch dressing powder
- 1/4 teaspoon of garlic powder
- 1/2 teaspoon of garlic pepper
- 1/2 cup of milk
- 1 large tomato, minced
- 1 can of sliced black olives (4.25 oz)
- 1 cup grated cheddar cheese

## INSTRUCTIONS:

**1.** Bring a large pot of lightly salted water to a boil; cook the rotini until tender but firm, about 8 minutes; drain.

**2.** Place the bacon in a frying pan over medium heat and cook until evenly browned. Drain and chop.

**3.** Combine mayonnaise, ranch dressing, garlic powder, and garlic pepper in a large bowl. Stir the milk until smooth.

**4.** Put the rotini, bacon, tomatoes, black olives, and cheese in a bowl and mix to cover with vinaigrette. Cover and put in the fridge for at least 1 hour.

**PER SERVING:** Calories 336 Fat 26.8 g Carbohydrates 14.9 g Protein 9.3 g

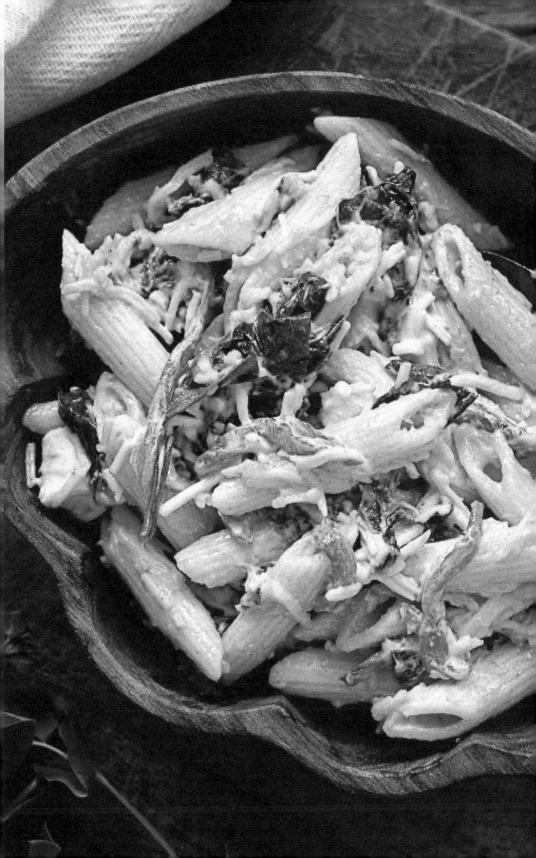

# Alfredo Peppered Shrimp

**Preparation time:** 15 minutes

**Cooking time:** 20 minutes

**Servings:** 6

## INGREDIENTS:

- [ ] 3 pounds penne
- [ ] 1/4 cup butter
- [ ] 2 tablespoons extra virgin olive oil
- [ ] 1 onion, diced
- [ ] 2 cloves of chopped garlic
- [ ] 1 red pepper, diced
- [ ] 1-pound portobello mushrooms, cubed
- [ ] 1 pound shrimp, peeled and thawed
- [ ] 1 jar of Alfredo sauce
- [ ] 1/2 cup of grated Romano cheese
- [ ] 1/2 cup of cream
- [ ] 1/4 cup chopped parsley
- [ ] 1 teaspoon cayenne pepper

salt and pepper to taste

## INSTRUCTIONS:

**1.** Bring a large pot of lightly salted water to a boil. Put the pasta and

cook for 8 to 10 minutes or until al dente; drain.

**2.** Meanwhile, melt the butter and olive oil in a pan over medium heat. Stir in the onion and cook until soft and translucent, about 2 minutes.

**3.** Stir in garlic, red pepper and mushrooms; cook over medium heat until soft, about 2 minutes longer.

**4.** Stir in the shrimp and fry until firm and pink, then add Alfredo sauce, Romano cheese and cream; bring to a boil, constantly stirring until thick, about 5 minutes.

**5.** Season with cayenne pepper, salt, and pepper to taste. Add the drained pasta to the sauce and sprinkle with chopped parsley.

**PER SERVING:** Calories 707 Fat 45 g Carbohydrates 50.6 g Protein 28.4 g

# Bow Ties with Sausages, Tomatoes & Cream

**Preparation time:** 15 minutes

**Cooking time:** 25 minutes

**Servings:** 6

## INGREDIENTS:

- [ ] 1 package of bowtie pasta
- [ ] 2 tablespoons of olive oil
- [ ] 1 pound of sweet Italian sausages, crumbled
- [ ] 1/2 teaspoon of red pepper flakes
- [ ] 1/2 cup diced onion
- [ ] 3 finely chopped garlic cloves
- [ ] 1 can of Italian tomatoes, drained and roughly chopped
- [ ] 1 1/2 cup whipped cream
- [ ] 1/2 teaspoon salt
- [ ] 3 tablespoons fresh parsley

## INSTRUCTIONS:

**1.** Bring a large pot of lightly salted water to a boil. Cook the pasta for 8 to 10 minutes in boiling water or until al dente; drain.

**2.** Heat the oil in a deep-frying pan over medium heat. Cook the sausages and chili flakes until the sausages are golden brown.

**3.** Stir in onion and garlic and cook until the onion is soft. Stir in the tomatoes, cream, and salt. Simmer until thickened, 8 to 10 minutes.

**4.** Add the pasta cooked in the sauce and heat. Sprinkle with

parsley.

**PER SERVING:** Calories 656 Fat 42.1 g Carbohydrates 50.9 g Protein

20.1 g

# Penne with Spicy Vodka Tomato Cream Sauce

**Preparation time:** 15 minutes

**Cooking time:** 25 minutes

**Servings:** 8

## INGREDIENTS:

- ☐ 1-pound uncooked penne
- ☐ 1/4 cup extra virgin olive oil
- ☐ 4 cloves finely chopped garlic
- ☐ 1/2 teaspoon crushed red pepper flakes
- ☐ 1 can of crushed tomatoes
- ☐ 3/4 teaspoon of salt
- ☐ 2 tablespoons of vodka
- ☐ 1/2 cup thick whipped cream
- ☐ 1/4 cup chopped fresh parsley
- ☐ 2 (3.5 ounces) sweet Italian sausage links

## INSTRUCTIONS:

**1.** Bring a large pan of lightly salted water to a boil. Put the pasta and cook for 8 to 10 minutes or until al dente; drain.

**2.** Heat the oil in a large frying pan over medium heat. Remove the casing from the sausage and add it to the pan.

**3.** Cook by browning the meat, add garlic and red pepper and cook, stirring until the garlic is golden brown. Add tomatoes and salt; boil. Lower the heat and simmer for 15 minutes.

41

**4.** Add vodka and cream and bring to a boil. Reduce the heat and add the pasta, mix for 1 minute. Stir in the fresh parsley and serve!

**PER SERVING:** Calories 435 Fat 18.4 g Carbohydrates 52.7 g Protein 13.3 g

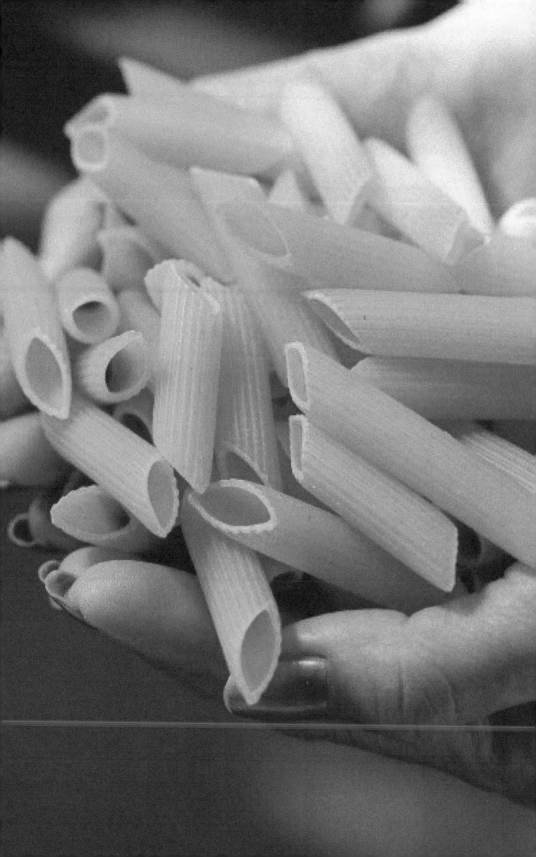

# Milanese Chicken

**Preparation time:** 15 minutes

**Cooking time:** 35 minutes

**Servings:** 4

## INGREDIENTS:

- ½ cup of sun-dried tomatoes, minced
- 1 cup of chicken broth, divided
- 1 cup thick cream
- 1 pound skinless and skinless chicken fillet
- 1 tablespoon butter
- 2 cloves of garlic, minced
- 2 tablespoons chopped fresh basil
- 8 grams of dry fettuccine
- salt and pepper to taste
- 2 tablespoons vegetable oil

## INSTRUCTIONS:

**1.** Once the butter is melted in a large pan over low heat, season with garlic and allow to simmer for 30 seconds. Add tomatoes and 3/4 cup chicken broth; and keep heating on a medium heat.

**2.** Once the liquid starts to boil, reduce the heat and simmer for about 10 minutes without a lid or until the tomatoes are soft. Add the cream and keep simmering until the sauce thickens.

**3.** Season with salt and pepper, the chicken on both sides. Heat oil in a large frying pan over medium-high heat and fry the chicken.

**4.** Press the chicken occasionally with a slotted spatula. Bake for about 4 minutes per side. Set aside; cover and keep warm. Discard the fat from the pan.

**5.** In the same pan, bring to a boil 1/4 cup chicken broth over medium heat. Reduce slightly and add to the cream sauce; stir in the basil and adjust the seasonings to taste.

**6.** Meanwhile, boil a large pan with lightly salted water. Add fettuccine and cook for about 8 to 10 minutes or until al dente; drain, transfer to a bowl and mix with 3 to 4 tablespoons of sauce.

**7.** Cut each chicken fillet into 2 or 3 diagonal slices. Heat the sauce carefully if necessary. Transfer the pasta to serving trays; garnish with chicken and sprinkle with cream sauce to serve.

**PER SERVING:** Calories 641 Fat 34.8 g Carbohydrates 47 g Protein 36.3 g

# One Pan Orecchiette Pasta

**Preparation time:** 15 minutes

**Cooking time:** 30 minutes

**Servings:** 2

## INGREDIENTS:

- [ ] 2 tablespoons olive oil
- [ ] 1/2 onion, diced
- [ ] salt to taste
- [ ] 8 grams of spicy Italian sausages
- [ ] 3 1/2 cups of low-sodium chicken broth, divided or as required
- [ ] 1 1/4 cup orecchiette pasta
- [ ] 1/2 cup chopped arugula
- [ ] 1/4 cup finely grated Parmigiano-Reggiano cheese

## INSTRUCTIONS:

**1.** Heat the olive oil in a deep-frying pan over medium heat. Cook and stir the onion with a pinch of salt until soft and golden brown, 5 to 7 minutes. Stir the sausages with onions, 5 to 7 minutes.

**2.** Pour 1 1/2 cup chicken stock into the sausage mixture and bring to a boil. Add the pasta to the orecchiette; boil and mix the pasta in a warm broth.

**3.** Add the remaining broth when the liquid is absorbed until the pasta is well cooked, and most of the broth is absorbed, about 15 minutes.

**4.** Stir in the sausage mixture. Spread the pasta in bowls and

sprinkle with Parmigiano-Reggiano cheese.

**PER SERVING:** Calories 662 Fat 39.1 g Carbohydrates 46.2 g Protein

31.2 g

# Rustic Pasta

**Preparation time:** 15 minutes

**Cooking time:** 30 minutes

**Servings:** 6

## INGREDIENTS:

- 1 pound of rotini or pasta fusilli
- 6 slices of bacon
- 1/2 cup of extra virgin olive oil
- 2 medium onions, minced
- 1 red pepper, minced
- 1/4 cup chopped parsley
- 4 cloves of garlic, minced
- Salt (optional)
- 1/2 teaspoon of crushed red pepper flakes
- 1 can (28 ounces) of yellow tomatoes, unsalted, coarsely
- chopped
- 1/2 cup black or green ripe seedless olives, sliced and drained

2 tablespoons drained capers

- 1/2 teaspoon dried oregano
- 1/2 cup grated Parmesan cheese

## INSTRUCTIONS:

**1.** Cook the pasta according to the instructions on the package. Meanwhile, fry bacon in a deep-frying pan until crispy. Drain the bacon on a paper towel; break into 1/2-inch pieces.

**2.** Discard the bacon juice from the pan; add the oil. Sauté onions in oil over medium heat for 5 minutes, stirring occasionally.

**3.** Add pepper, parsley, garlic, and pepper flakes; cook for 2 minutes. Add tomatoes and reserved bacon; simmer 10 minutes, stirring occasionally.

**4.** Stir olives and oregano; simmer for 2 minutes. Season with salt, if desired. Drain the pasta; mix with the sauce and cheese.

**PER SERVING:** Calories 593 Fat 27.6 g Carbohydrates 68.6 g Protein 17.8 g

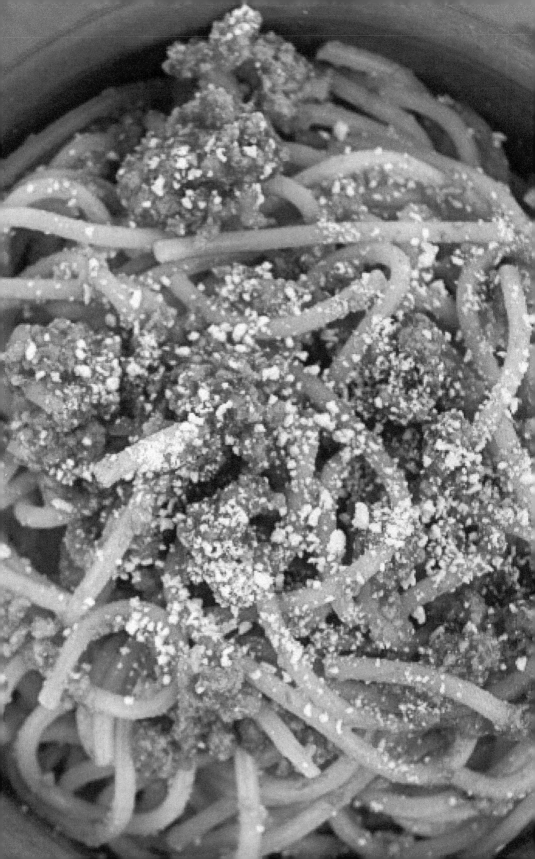

# Creamy Cajun Chicken Pasta

**Preparation time:** 15 minutes

**Cooking time:** 20 minutes

**Servings:** 2

## INGREDIENTS:

- [ ] 4 oz linguine
- [ ] 2 boneless chicken fillets, skinless, cut into thin strips
- [ ] 2 teaspoons Cajun herbs
- [ ] 2 tablespoons butter
- [ ] 1 green pepper, minced
- [ ] ½ red pepper, minced
- [ ] 4 fresh chopped mushrooms
- [ ] 1 chopped green onion
- [ ] 1 ½ cups thick cream
- [ ] ¼ teaspoon dried basil
- [ ] ¼ teaspoon lemon pepper
- [ ] ¼ teaspoon salt
- [ ] 1 teaspoon garlic powder

1/8 teaspoon ground black pepper

- [ ] 2 tablespoons grated Parmesan cheese

## INSTRUCTIONS:

**1.** Bring a large pot of lightly salted water to a boil. Add linguini and

cook for 8 to 10 minutes or until al dente; drain. In the meantime, put the chicken and Cajun herbs in a bowl and mix to coat.

**2.** Bake chicken in butter in a large frying pan over medium heat for 5 to 7 minutes. Add green and red peppers, chopped mushrooms, and green onions; cook 2 to 3 minutes.

**3.** Reduce the heat and stir in the whipped cream. Season the sauce with basil, lemon pepper, salt, garlic powder, and ground black pepper and heat.

**4.** Mix the linguini with the sauce in a large bowl. Sprinkle with grated Parmesan cheese.

**PER SERVING:** Calories 1109 Fat 82.2 g Carbohydrates 53.7 g Protein 42.7 g

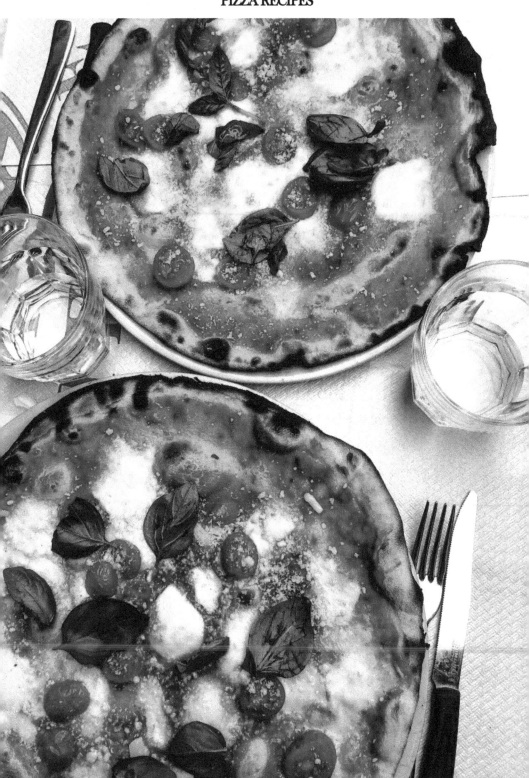

# Balsamic-Glazed Pizza with Arugula & Olives

**Preparation time:** 1 hour & 20 minutes

**Cooking time:** 20 minutes

**Servings:** 4

## INGREDIENTS:

- [ ] 2 cups flour
- [ ] 1 cup lukewarm water
- [ ] 1 pinch of sugar
- [ ] 1 tsp active dry yeast
- [ ] 2 tbsp olive oil
- [ ] 2 tbsp honey
- [ ] ½ cup balsamic vinegar
- [ ] 4 cups arugula
- [ ] Salt and black pepper to taste
- [ ] 1 cup mozzarella cheese, grated
- [ ] ¾ tsp dried oregano
- [ ] 6 black olives, drained

## INSTRUCTIONS:

**1.** Sift the flour and ¾ tsp salt in a bowl and stir in yeast. Mix lukewarm water, olive oil, and sugar in another bowl. Add the wet mixture to the dry mixture and whisk until you obtain a soft dough.

**2.** Place the dough on a lightly floured work surface and knead it thoroughly for 4-5 minutes until elastic. Transfer the dough to a greased bowl.

**3.** Cover with cling film and leave to rise for 50-60 minutes in a warm place until doubled in size. Roll out the dough to a thickness of around 12 inches.

**4.** Place the balsamic vinegar and honey in a saucepan over medium heat and simmer for 5 minutes until syrupy. Preheat oven to 390 F.

**5.** Transfer the pizza crust to a baking sheet and sprinkle with oregano and mozzarella cheese; bake for 10-15 minutes.

**6.** Remove the pizza from the oven and top with arugula. Sprinkle with balsamic glaze and black olives and serve.

**PER SERVING:** Calories 350 Fat 15.4g Carbs 47.1g Protein 6.4g

# Pepperoni Fat Head Pizza

**Preparation time:** 1 hour & 20 minutes

**Cooking time:** 15 minutes

**Servings:** 4

## INGREDIENTS:

- ☐ 2 cups flour
- ☐ 1 cup lukewarm water
- ☐ 1 pinch of sugar
- ☐ 1 tsp active dry yeast
- ☐ ¾ tsp salt
- ☐ 2 tbsp olive oil
- ☐ 1 tsp dried oregano
- ☐ 2 cups mozzarella cheese
- ☐ 1 cup sliced pepperoni

## INSTRUCTIONS:

**1.** Sift the flour and salt in a bowl and stir in yeast. Mix lukewarm water, olive oil, and sugar in another bowl. Add the wet mixture to the dry mixture and whisk until you obtain a soft dough.

**2.** Place the dough on a lightly floured work surface and knead it thoroughly for 4-5 minutes until elastic. Transfer the dough to a greased bowl.

**3.** Cover with cling film and leave to rise for 50-60 minutes in a warm place until doubled in size. Roll out the dough to a thickness of around 12 inches.

**4.** Preheat oven to 400 F. Line a round pizza pan with parchment paper. Spread the dough on the pizza pan and top with the mozzarella cheese, oregano, and pepperoni slices.

**5.** Bake in the oven for 15 minutes or until the cheese melts. Remove the pizza, slice and serve.

**PER SERVING:** Calories 229 Fats 7.1g Carbs 0.4g Protein 36.4g

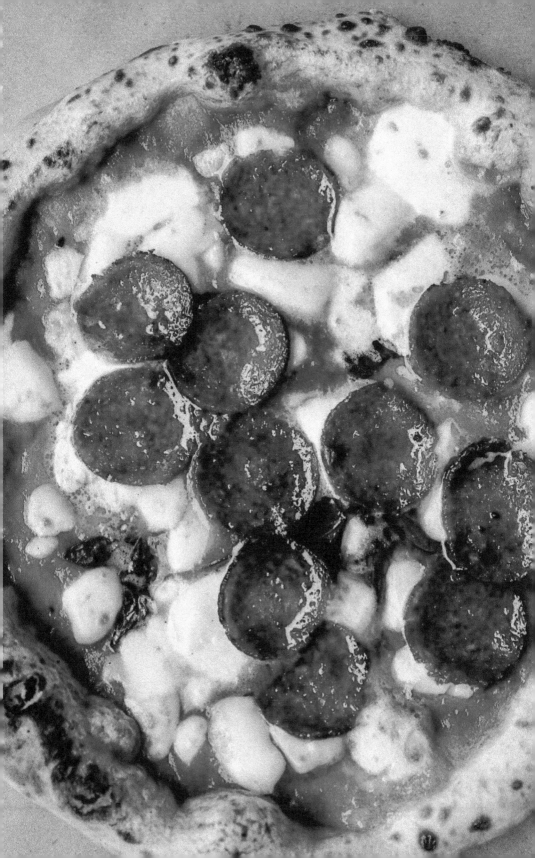

# Extra Cheesy Pizza

**Preparation time:** 15 minutes

**Cooking time:** 28 minutes

**Servings:** 4

## INGREDIENTS:

For the crust:

- ☐ ½ cup almond flour
- ☐ ¼ tsp salt
- ☐ 2 tbsp ground psyllium husk
- ☐ 1 tbsp olive oil
- ☐ 1 cup lukewarm water

For the topping

- ☐ ½ cup sugar-free pizza sauce
- ☐ 1 cup sliced mozzarella cheese
- ☐ 1 cup grated mozzarella cheese
- ☐ 3 tbsp grated Parmesan cheese
- ☐ 2 tsp Italian seasoning

## INSTRUCTIONS:

**1.** Preheat the oven to 400 F. Line a baking sheet with parchment paper. In a medium bowl, mix the almond flour, salt, psyllium powder, olive oil, and lukewarm water until dough forms.

**2.** Spread the mixture on the pizza pan and bake in the oven until crusty, 10 minutes. When ready, remove the crust and spread the pizza sauce on top.

**3.** Add the sliced mozzarella, grated mozzarella, Parmesan cheese, and Italian seasoning. Bake in the oven for 18 minutes or until the cheeses melt. Serve warm.

**PER SERVING:** Calories 193 Fats 10.2g Carbs 3.2g Protein 19.5g

# Spanish-Style Pizza de Jamon

**Preparation time:** 1 hour & 15 minutes

**Cooking time:** 15 minutes

**Servings:** 4

## INGREDIENTS:

For the crust:

- ☐ 2 cups flour
- ☐ 1 cup lukewarm water
- ☐ 1 pinch of sugar
- ☐ 1 tsp active dry yeast
- ☐ ¾ tsp salt
- ☐ 2 tbsp olive oil

For the topping:

- ☐ ½ cup tomato sauce
- ☐ ½ cup sliced mozzarella cheese
- ☐ 4 oz jamon serrano, sliced
- ☐ 7 fresh basil leaves

## INSTRUCTIONS:

**1.** Sift the flour and salt in a bowl and stir in yeast. Mix lukewarm water, olive oil, and sugar in another bowl. Add the wet mixture to the dry mixture and whisk until you obtain a soft dough.

**2.** Place the dough on a lightly floured work surface and knead it thoroughly for 4-5 minutes until elastic. Transfer the dough to a greased bowl.

**3.** Cover with cling film and leave to rise for 50-60 minutes in a warm place until doubled in size. Roll out the dough to a thickness of around 12 inches.

**4.** Preheat the oven to 400 F. Line a pizza pan with parchment paper. Spread the tomato sauce on the crust.

**5.** Arrange the mozzarella slices on the sauce and then the jamon serrano. Bake for 15 minutes or until the cheese melts. Remove from the oven and top with the basil. Slice and serve warm.

**PER SERVING:** Calories 160 Fats 6.2g Carbs 0.5g Protein 21.9g

# Spicy & Smoky Pizza

**Preparation time:** 1 hour & 15 minutes

**Cooking time:** 20 minutes

**Servings:** 4

## INGREDIENTS:

For the crust:

- ☐ 2 cups flour
- ☐ 1 cup lukewarm water
- ☐ 1 pinch of sugar
- ☐ 1 tsp active dry yeast
- ☐ ¾ tsp salt
- ☐ 2 tbsp olive oil

For the topping:

- ☐ 1 tbsp olive oil
- ☐ 1 cup sliced chorizo
- ☐ ¼ cup sugar-free marinara sauce
- ☐ 1 cup sliced smoked mozzarella cheese
- ☐ 1 jalapeño pepper, deseeded and sliced
- ☐ ¼ red onion, thinly sliced

## INSTRUCTIONS:

**1.** Sift the flour and salt in a bowl and stir in yeast. Mix lukewarm water, olive oil, and sugar in another bowl. Add the wet mixture to the dry mixture and whisk until you obtain a soft dough.

**2.** Place the dough on a lightly floured work surface and knead it thoroughly for 4-5 minutes until elastic. Transfer the dough to a greased bowl.

**3.** Cover with cling film and leave to rise for 50-60 minutes in a warm place until doubled in size. Roll out the dough to a thickness of around 12 inches.

**4.** Preheat the oven to 400 F. Line a pizza pan with parchment paper. Heat the olive oil and cook the chorizo until brown, 5 minutes.

**5.** Spread the marinara sauce on the crust, top with the mozzarella cheese, chorizo, jalapeño pepper, and onion.

**6.** Bake in the oven until the cheese melts, 15 minutes. Remove from the oven, slice, and serve warm.

**PER SERVING:** Calories 302 Fats 17g Carbs 1.4g Protein 31.6g

# Turkey Pizza with Pesto Topping

**Preparation time:** 15 minutes

**Cooking time:** 30 minutes

**Servings:** 4

## INGREDIENTS:

Pizza Crust:

- ☐ 3 cups flour
- ☐ 3 tbsp olive oil
- ☐ 1/3 tsp salt
- ☐ 3 large eggs

Pesto Chicken Topping:

- ☐ ½ lb. turkey ham, chopped
- ☐ 2 tbsp cashew nuts
- ☐ Salt and black pepper to taste
- ☐ 1 ½ tbsp olive oil
- ☐ 1 green bell pepper, seeded and sliced
- ☐ 1 ½ cups basil pesto
- ☐ 1 cup mozzarella cheese, grated

1 ½ tbsp Parmesan cheese, grated

- ☐ 1½ tbsp fresh basil leaves
- ☐ A pinch of red pepper flakes

## INSTRUCTIONS:

**1.** In a bowl, mix flour, 3 tbsp of olive oil, salt, and eggs until a dough form. Mold the dough into a ball and place it in between two full parchment papers on a flat surface.

**2.** Roll it out into a circle of a ¼ -inch thickness. After, slide the pizza dough into the pizza pan and remove the parchment paper. Place the pizza pan in the oven and bake the dough for 20 minutes at 350°F.

**3.** Once the pizza bread is ready, remove it from the oven, fold and seal the extra inch of dough at its edges to make a crust around it.

**4.** Apply 2/3 of the pesto on it and sprinkle half of the mozzarella cheese too. Toss the chopped turkey ham in the remaining pesto and spread it on top of the pizza.

**5.** Sprinkle with the remaining mozzarella, bell peppers, and cashew nuts and put the pizza back in the oven to bake for 9 minutes.

**6.** When it is ready, remove from the oven to cool slightly, garnish with the basil leaves and sprinkle with parmesan cheese and red pepper flakes. Slice and serve.

**PER SERVING:** Calories 684 Fat 54g Carbs 22g Protein 31.5g

# Baby Spinach Pizza with Sweet Onion

**Preparation time:** 1 hour & 15 minutes

**Cooking time:** 53 minutes

**Servings:** 4

**INGREDIENTS:**

For the crust:

- ☐ 2 cups flour
- ☐ 1 cup lukewarm water
- ☐ 1 pinch of sugar
- ☐ 1 tsp active dry yeast
- ☐ ¾ tsp salt
- ☐ 2 tbsp olive oil

For the caramelized onion:

- ☐ 1 onion, sliced
- ☐ 1 tsp sugar
- ☐ 2 tbsp olive oil
- ☐ ½ tsp salt

For the pizza:

- ☐ ¼ cup shaved Pecorino Romano cheese
- ☐ 2 tbsp olive oil
- ☐ ½ cup grated mozzarella cheese
- ☐ 1 cup baby spinach
- ☐ ¼ cup chopped fresh basil leaves
- ☐ ½ red bell pepper, sliced

## INSTRUCTIONS:

**1.** Sift the flour and salt in a bowl and stir in yeast. Mix lukewarm water, olive oil, and sugar in another bowl. Add the wet mixture to the dry mixture and whisk until you obtain a soft dough.

**2.** Place the dough on a lightly floured work surface and knead it thoroughly for 4-5 minutes until elastic. Transfer the dough to a greased bowl.

**3.** Cover with cling film and leave to rise for 50-60 minutes in a warm place until doubled in size. Roll out the dough to a thickness of around 12 inches.

**4.** Warm olive oil in a skillet over medium heat and sauté onion with salt and sugar for 3 minutes. Lower the heat and brown for 20-35 minutes until caramelized. Preheat oven to 390 F.

**5.** Transfer the pizza crust to a baking sheet. Drizzle the crust with olive oil and top with onion. Cover with bell pepper and mozzarella. Bake for 10-15 minutes. Serve topped with baby spinach, basil, and Pecorino cheese.

**PER SERVING:** Calories 399 Fat 22.7g Carbs 42.9g Protein 8.1g

# Italian Mushroom Pizza

**Preparation time:** 1 hour & 15 minutes

**Cooking time:** 25 minutes

**Servings:** 4

## INGREDIENTS:

For the crust:

- ☐ 2 cups flour
- ☐ 1 cup lukewarm water
- ☐ 1 pinch of sugar
- ☐ 1 tsp active dry yeast
- ☐ ¾ tsp salt
- ☐ 2 tbsp olive oil

For the topping:

- ☐ 1 tsp olive oil
- ☐ 2 medium cremini mushrooms, sliced
- ☐ 1 garlic clove, minced
- ☐ ½ cup sugar-free tomato sauce
- ☐ 1 tsp sugar
- ☐ 1 bay leaf
- ☐ 1 tsp dried oregano
- ☐ 1tsp dried basil
- ☐ Salt and black pepper to taste
- ☐ ½ cup grated mozzarella cheese
- ☐ ½ cup grated Parmesan cheese

☐  6 black olives, pitted and sliced

## INSTRUCTIONS:

**1.** Sift the flour and salt in a bowl and stir in yeast. Mix lukewarm water, olive oil, and sugar in another bowl. Add the wet mixture to the dry mixture and whisk until you obtain a soft dough.

**2.** Place the dough on a lightly floured work surface and knead it thoroughly for 4-5 minutes until elastic. Transfer the dough to a greased bowl.

**3.** Cover with cling film and leave to rise for 50-60 minutes in a warm place until doubled in size. Roll out the dough to a thickness of around 12 inches.

**4.** Preheat the oven to 400 F. Line a pizza pan with parchment paper. Heat the olive oil in a medium skillet and sauté the mushrooms until softened, 5 minutes. Stir in the garlic and cook until fragrant, 30 seconds.

**5.** Mix in the tomato sauce, sugar, bay leaf, oregano, basil, salt, and black pepper. Cook for 2 minutes and turn the heat off.

**6.** Spread the sauce on the crust, top with the mozzarella and Parmesan cheeses, and then, the olives. Bake in the oven until the cheese's melts, 15 minutes. Remove the pizza, slice, and serve warm.

**PER SERVING:** Calories 203 Fats 8.6g Carbs 2.6g Protein 24.3g

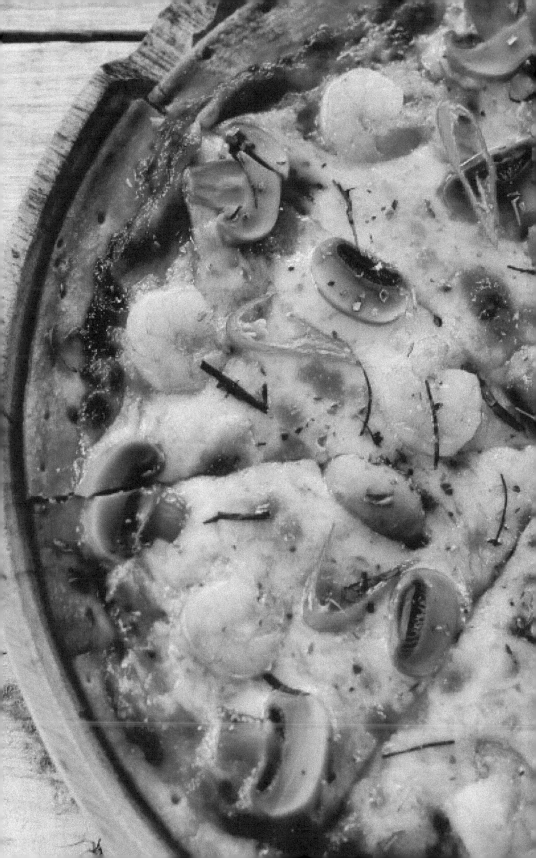

# Broccoli-Pepper Pizza

**Preparation time:** 15 minutes

**Cooking time:** 20 minutes

**Servings:** 4

## INGREDIENTS:

For the crust:

- ☐ ½ cup almond flour
- ☐ ¼ tsp salt
- ☐ 2 tbsp ground psyllium husk
- ☐ 1 tbsp olive oil
- ☐ 1 cup lukewarm water

For the topping:

- ☐ 1 tbsp olive oil
- ☐ 1 cup sliced fresh mushrooms
- ☐ 1 white onion, thinly sliced
- ☐ 3 cups broccoli florets
- ☐ 4 garlic cloves, minced
- ☐ ½ cup pizza sauce
- ☐ 4 tomatoes, sliced
- ☐ 1 ½ cup grated mozzarella cheese
- ☐ ½ cup grated Parmesan cheese

## INSTRUCTIONS:

**1.** Preheat the oven to 400 F. Line a baking sheet with parchment

paper. In a bowl, mix the almond flour, salt, psyllium powder, olive oil, and lukewarm water until dough forms.

**2.** Spread the mixture on the pizza pan and bake in the oven until crusty, 10 minutes. When ready, remove the crust and allow cooling.

**3.** Heat olive oil in a skillet and sauté the mushrooms, onion, garlic, and broccoli until softened, 5 minutes.

**4.** Spread the pizza sauce on the crust and top with the broccoli mixture, tomato, mozzarella and Parmesan cheeses. Bake for 5 minutes.

**PER SERVING:** Calories 180 Fats 9g Carbs 3.6g Protein 17g

# White Pizza with Prosciutto and Arugula

**Preparation Time:** 10 minutes

**Cooking Time:** 15 minutes

**Servings:** 6

## INGREDIENTS:

- ☐ 1 lb. prepared pizza dough
- ☐ ½ cup ricotta cheese
- ☐ 1 tbsp. garlic, minced
- ☐ 1 cup grated mozzarella cheese
- ☐ 3 oz. prosciutto, thinly sliced
- ☐ ½ cup fresh arugula
- ☐ ½ tsp. freshly ground black pepper

## INSTRUCTIONS:

**1.** Preheat the oven to 450°F. Roll out the pizza dough on a floured

surface. Put the pizza dough on a parchment-lined baking sheet

or pizza sheet. Put the dough in the oven and bake for 8 minutes.

**2.** In a small bowl, mix together the ricotta, garlic, and mozzarella.

Remove the pizza dough from the oven and spread the cheese

mixture over the top.

**3.** Bake for another 5 to 6 minutes. Top the pizza with prosciutto,

arugula, and pepper; serve warm.

**PER SERVING:** Calories: 273 Protein: 12.3g Carbs: 34g Fat: 11g

# Za'atar Pizza

**Preparation Time:** 10 minutes

**Cooking Time:** 15 minutes

**Servings:** 5

## INGREDIENTS:

- ☐ 1 sheet puff pastry
- ☐ ¼ cup extra-virgin olive oil
- ☐ 1/3 cup za'atar seasoning

## INSTRUCTIONS:

**1.** Preheat the oven to 350°F. Put the puff pastry on a parchmentlined baking sheet. Cut the pastry into desired slices.

**2.** Brush the pastry with olive oil. Sprinkle with the za'atar. Put the pastry in the oven and bake for 10 to 12 minutes or until edges are lightly browned and puffed up. Serve warm or at room temperature.

**PER SERVING:** Calories: 153 Protein: 10.3g Carbs: 21g Fat: 10g

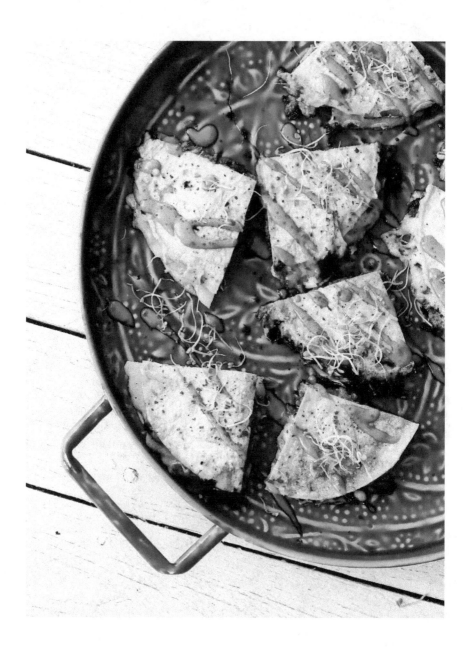

# Broccoli Cheese Burst Pizza

**Preparation Time:** 20 minutes

**Cooking Time:** 5 minutes

**Servings:** 6

## INGREDIENTS:

- ☐ 1 cup mozzarella cheese, shredded
- ☐ 2/3 cup ricotta cheese
- ☐ 2 tsp. avocado oil
- ☐ 1 large whole-wheat pizza crust
- ☐ ¼ cup basil, chopped
- ☐ 1 ½ cups broccoli florets, chopped
- ☐ ½ tsp. garlic powder
- ☐ Cornmeal (for dusting)
- ☐ 1 ½ cups corn kernels
- ☐ Ground black pepper and salt, to taste

## INSTRUCTIONS:

**1.** Preheat your oven at 400°F. Take a baking sheet, line it with parchment paper. Grease it with some avocado oil. Spread some cornmeal over the baking sheet

**2.** In a mixing bowl, combine the corn, broccoli, ricotta, mozzarella, scallions, garlic powder, basil, black pepper and salt.

**3.** Place the pizza crust on the baking sheet. Add the topping mixture on top and bake until the top is light brown, for 12-15

minutes. Slice and serve warm!

**PER SERVING:** Calories 417 Fat 11g Carbs 53g Protein 19g

# Mozzarella Bean Pizza

**Preparation Time:** 10 minutes

**Cooking Time:** 15 minutes

**Servings:** 6

## INGREDIENTS:

- ☐ 2 tbsp. cornmeal
- ☐ 1 cup mozzarella
- ☐ 1/3 cup barbecue sauce
- ☐ 1 roma tomato, diced
- ☐ 1 cup black beans
- ☐ 1 cup corn kernels
- ☐ 1 medium whole-wheat pizza crust

## INSTRUCTIONS:

**1.** Preheat your oven at 400°F. Take a baking sheet, line it with parchment paper. Grease it with some avocado oil. Spread some cornmeal over the baking sheet.

**2.** In a bowl, mix together the tomatoes, corn and beans. Place the pizza crust on the baking sheet.

**3.** Spread the sauce on top; add the topping, and top with the cheese and bake until the cheese melts and the crust edges are golden-brown for 12-15 minutes. Slice and serve warm.

**PER SERVING:** Calories 223 Fat 14g Carbs 41g Protein 8g

# Pizza Dough Without Yeast in Milk

**Preparation Time:** 5 minutes

**Cooking Time:** 1 hour

**Servings:** 5

## INGREDIENTS:

- [ ] Wheat flour 2 cups
- [ ] Milk 125 ml
- [ ] Salt 1 tsp.
- [ ] Chicken egg 2 pieces
- [ ] Sunflower oil 2 tbsp.

## INSTRUCTIONS:

**1.** Making pizza dough without yeast in milk is quite simple. The recipe is designed to prepare a dough, which is enough for two, but only large, baking sheets.

**2.** Combine flour and salt in one bowl. And in the second butter, milk and eggs, mix well and combine the contents of two bowls in one large container.

**3.** Wait a few minutes for the whole liquid consistency to soak in the flour, and start mixing the dough. It will take about 15 minutes. Dough, in finished form, should be elastic, soft and smooth.

**4.** Then you need to take a kitchen towel, of course clean, and soak it in water. As a result, it should be moist, but not wet. Excess fluid must be squeezed out. Wrap the dough in a towel, leave to lie down for 20 minutes.

**5.** After waiting for the set time, remove the dough and, sprinkling flour on the countertop, roll out, but only very thinly.

**6.** Place it on a baking sheet and lay out the filling prepared according to your taste preferences. As a result, the finished dough will have an effect that is easy, of course, of puff pastry and has a crispy taste.

**PER SERVING:** Calories: 453 Protein: 10.3g Carbs: 30.4g Fat: 14.3g

# Ideal Pizza Dough (On A Large Baking Sheet)

**Preparation Time:** 10 minutes

**Cooking Time:** 1 hour

**Servings:** 5

## INGREDIENTS:

- ☐ Wheat flour 13 oz.
- ☐ Salt 1.5 tsp.
- ☐ Dry yeast 1,799 tsp.
- ☐ Sugar 1 tsp.
- ☐ Water 200 ml
- ☐ 1 tbsp. olive oil
- ☐ Dried Basil 1.5 tsp.

## INSTRUCTIONS:

**1.** We cultivate yeast in warm water. There you can add a spoonful of sugar, so the yeast will begin to work faster. Leave them for 10 minutes.

**2.** Sift the flour through a sieve (leave 2 oz. for the future) in a deep bowl. Add salt, basil, mix. Pour water with yeast into the cavity in the flour and mix thoroughly with a fork.

**3.** Somewhere in the middle of the process, when the dough becomes less than one whole, add olive oil. When the dough is ready, cover with a damp towel and put in heat for 30 minutes.

**4.** Now just lay it on a flour dusted surface and roll out the future pizza to a thickness of 2-3 mm.

**5.** The main rule of pizza is the maximum possible temperature, minimum time. Therefore, feel free to set the highest temperature that is available in your oven.

**PER SERVING:** Calories: 193 Protein: 10.3g Carbs: 34g Fat: 9.3g

# Vegetable Oil Pizza Dough

**Preparation Time:** 10 minutes

**Cooking Time:** 1 hour

**Servings:** 3

## INGREDIENTS:

- ☐ Wheat flour 1 cup
- ☐ Water 1 cup
- ☐ Salt to taste
- ☐ Vegetable oil 1 tbsp.
- ☐ Dry yeast 10 g

## INSTRUCTIONS:

**1.** We mix water and yeast, leave for 40 minutes so that they disperse. You can add a tablespoon of sugar.

**2.** Then pour in the oil, add the flour; knead well and put in a warm place to increase the volume by 2 times.

**PER SERVING:** Calories: 223 Protein: 10.3g Carbs: 9.4g Fat: 5.3g

# Pizza Dough on Yogurt

**Preparation Time:** 10 minutes

**Cooking Time:** 30 minutes

**Servings:** 5

## INGREDIENTS:

- ☐ Natural yogurt 9 oz.
- ☐ Vegetable oil 5 tbsp.
- ☐ ½ tsp. salt
- ☐ Wheat flour 2.5 cups
- ☐ Baking powder 1 tsp.

## INSTRUCTIONS:

**1.** Mix flour, baking powder and salt. Add yogurt and butter, mix everything thoroughly. Preheat the oven to 190 ° C.

**2.** Lubricate the pan with oil. Roll the dough very thinly and transfer to a baking sheet. Put the filling to taste. Bake for 10-15 minutes.

**PER SERVING:** Calories: 336 Protein: 10.3g Carbs: 24g Fat: 13.3g

# Eggplant Pizza

**Preparation Time:** 10 minutes

**Cooking Time:** 30 minutes

**Servings:** 6

## INGREDIENTS:

- ☐ Eggplants (1 large or 2 medium)
- ☐ Olive oil (.33 cup)
- ☐ Black pepper & salt (as desired)
- ☐ Marinara sauce - store-bought/homemade (1.25 cups)
- ☐ Shredded mozzarella cheese (1.5 cups)
- ☐ Cherry tomatoes (2 cups - halved)
- ☐ Torn basil leaves (.5 cup)

## INSTRUCTIONS:

**1.** Heat the oven to reach 400°F. Prepare a baking sheet with a layer of parchment baking paper.

**2.** Slice the end/ends off of the eggplant and them it into ¾-inch slices. Arrange the slices on the prepared sheet and brush both sides with olive oil. Dust with pepper and salt to your liking.

**3.** Roast the eggplant until tender (10 to 12 min.).

**4.** Transfer the tray from the oven and add two tbsp. of sauce on top of each section. Top it off with the mozzarella and three to five tomato pieces on top.

**5.** Bake it until the cheese is melted. The tomatoes should begin to blister in about five to seven more minutes. Take the tray from the oven. Serve hot and garnish with a dusting of basil.

**PER SERVING:** Protein: 8 g Fat: 20 g Carbs: 25 g Calories: 257

# Mediterranean Whole Wheat Pizza

**Preparation Time:** 5 minutes

**Cooking Time:** 25 minutes

**Servings:** 4

## INGREDIENTS:

- ☐ Whole-wheat pizza crust (1)
- ☐ Basil pesto (4 oz. jar)
- ☐ Artichoke hearts (.5 cup)
- ☐ Kalamata olives (2 tbsp.)
- ☐ Pepperoncini (2 tbsp. drained)
- ☐ Feta cheese (.25 cup)

## INSTRUCTIONS:

**1.** Program the oven to 450°F. Drain and pull the artichokes to pieces. Slice/chop the pepperoncini and olives.

**2.** Arrange the pizza crust onto a floured work surface and cover it using pesto. Arrange the artichoke, pepperoncini slices, and olives over the pizza. Lastly, crumble and add the feta.

**3.** Bake in the hot oven until the cheese has melted, and it has a crispy crust or 10-12 minutes.

**PER SERVING:** Calories: 277 Protein: 9.7 g Carbs: 24 g Fat: 18.6 g

# Fruit Pizza

**Preparation time**: 15 minutes

**Cooking time:** 0 minutes

**Servings:** 4

## INGREDIENTS:

- ☐  4 watermelon slices
- ☐  1 oz blueberries
- ☐  2 oz goat cheese, crumbled
- ☐  1 teaspoon fresh parsley, chopped

## INSTRUCTIONS:

**1.** Put the watermelon slices in the plate in one layer. Then sprinkle

them with blueberries, goat cheese, and fresh parsley.

**PER SERVING:** Calories 69 Protein 4.4g Carbohydrates 1.4g Fat 5.1g

# Sprouts Pizza

**Preparation time:** 15 minutes

**Cooking time:** 15 minutes

**Servings:** 6

## INGREDIENTS:

- 4 oz wheat flour, whole grain
- 2 tablespoons olive oil
- ¼ teaspoon baking powder
- 5 oz chicken fillet, boiled
- 2 oz Mozzarella cheese, shredded
- 1 tomato, chopped
- 2 oz bean sprouts

## INSTRUCTIONS:

**1.** Make the pizza crust: mix wheat flour, olive oil, baking powder, and knead the dough. Roll it up in the shape of pizza crust and transfer in the pizza mold.

**2.** Then sprinkle it with chopped tomato, shredded chicken, and Mozzarella. Bake the pizza at 365F for 15 minutes. Sprinkle the cooked pizza with bean sprouts and cut into servings.

**PER SERVING:** Calories 184 Protein 11.9g Carbohydrates 15.6g Fat 8.2g

# Cheese Pinwheels

**Preparation time:** 15 minutes

**Cooking time:** 25 minutes

**Servings:** 6

## INGREDIENTS:

- ☐ 1 teaspoon chili flakes
- ☐ ½ teaspoon dried cilantro
- ☐ 1 egg, beaten
- ☐ 1 teaspoon cream cheese
- ☐ 1 oz Cheddar cheese, grated
- ☐ 6 oz pizza dough

## INSTRUCTIONS:

**1.** Roll up the pizza dough and cut into 6 squares. Sprinkle the dough with dried cilantro, cream cheese, and Cheddar cheese.

**2.** Roll the dough in the shape of pinwheels, brush with beaten egg and bake in the preheated to 365F oven for 25 minutes or until the pinwheels are light brown.

**PER SERVING:** Calories 16 Protein 3.8g Carbohydrates 12.1g Fat 11.2g

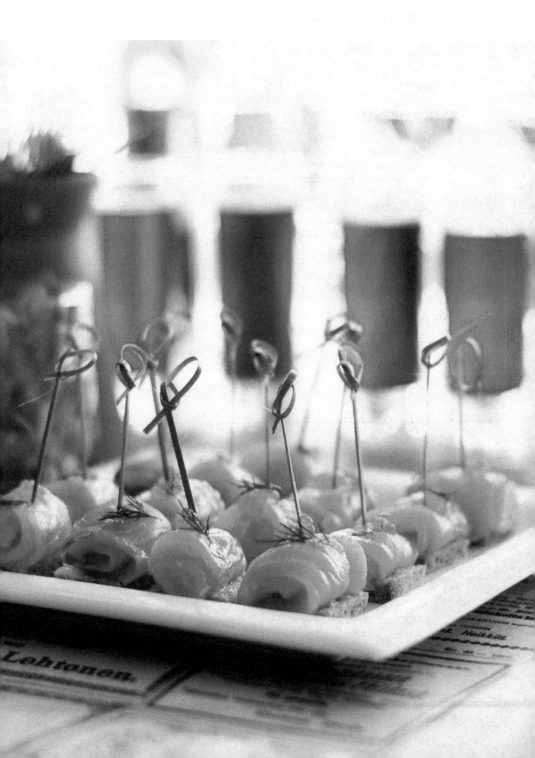

# Tomato Olive Salsa

**Preparation time:** 15 minutes

**Cooking Time:** 5 Minutes

**Servings:** 4

## INGREDIENTS:

- 2 cups olives, pitted and chopped
- 1/4 cup fresh parsley, chopped
- 1/4 cup fresh basil, chopped
- 2 tbsp green onion, chopped
- 1 cup grape tomatoes, halved
- 1 tbsp olive oil
- 1 tbsp vinegar
- Pepper
- Salt

## INSTRUCTIONS:

**1.** Add all ingredients into the inner pot of pot and stir well.

Seal pot with lid and cook on high for 5 minutes.

**2.** Once done, allow to release pressure naturally for 5 minutes then release remaining using quick release. Remove lid. Stir well and serve.

**PER SERVING:** Calories 119 Fat 10.8 g Carbohydrates 6.5 g Protein 1.2 g

# Thin-Crust Flatbread

**Preparation time:** 15 minutes

**Cooking time:** 25 minutes

**Servings:** 2

## INGREDIENTS:

- [ ] 2 cup all-purpose flour
- [ ] ¾ cup lukewarm water
- [ ] 1 teaspoon instant yeast
- [ ] 1 ½ teaspoon salt
- [ ] 1 tablespoon olive oil
- [ ] 1 garlic clove, crushed
- [ ] ¼ teaspoon sea salt
- [ ] ½ tomato, thinly sliced
- [ ] ¼ yellow beet, thinly sliced
- [ ] ½ Meyer lemon, thinly sliced
- [ ] ¼ potato, thinly sliced
- [ ] 1 radish, thinly sliced
- [ ] ½ burrata mozzarella ball, dotted all over flatbread
- [ ] 1 tablespoon fresh tarragon, chopped

## INSTRUCTIONS:

**1.** Mix yeast and water in a bowl and stir to dissolve the yeast. Add salt and flour to the bowl and mix well.

**2.** Turn the dough onto a clear surface. Knead well for 5 minutes. If dough is sticky, add 1 tablespoon flour at a time. Let the dough rise for 1 ½ hour. Cover with a bowl. Preheat the oven to 375F.

**3.** Roll out the flatbread. Brush olive oil over it. Rub crushed garlic over it. Sprinkle with sea salt. Lay toppings over it as you like.

**4.** Dollop cheese over it. Sprinkle with pinches of salt. Place in the oven and bake for 25 minutes. Top with tarragon. Serve.

**PER SERVING:** Calories: 150 Carbs: 27g Fat: 2g Protein: 7g

# Smoked Salmon Goat Cheese Endive Bites

**Preparation time:** 15 minutes

**Cooking time:** 0 minutes

**Servings:** 4

## INGREDIENTS:

- ☐ 1 package herbed goat cheese
- ☐ 3 endive heads
- ☐ 1 package smoked salmon

## INSTRUCTIONS:

**1.** Pull the leaves apart from endives and cut the ends off of them.

Add goat cheese to endive leaves. Add salmon slices on top of

the goat cheese.Serve.

**PER SERVING:** Calories: 46 Carbs: 1g Fat: 3g Protein: 3g

# Hummus Peppers

**Preparation time:** 15 minutes

**Cooking time:** 0 minutes

**Servings:** 12

## INGREDIENTS:

- ☐ 6 baby bell peppers, halved lengthwise
- ☐ 10 oz. hummus
- ☐ ¼ cup kalamata olives, pitted and chopped
- ☐ ¼ cup reduced fat crumbled feta
- ☐ parsley

## INSTRUCTIONS:

**1.** Place sliced bell peppers in a plate and add 2 tablespoons of

hummus to each. Add feta, olives and parsley. Serve.

**PER SERVING:** Calories: 70 Carbs: 4g Fat: 5g Protein: 2g

# Loaded Mediterranean Hummus

**Preparation time:** 15 minutes

**Cooking time:** 0 minutes

**Servings:** 2 cups

## INGREDIENTS:

- ☐ 1 tablespoon olive oil
- ☐ 2 cups hummus
- ☐ 1 teaspoon paprika
- ☐ 1 cup olives, sliced
- ☐ ½ red bell pepper, sliced
- ☐ 2 tablespoon pine nuts
- ☐ 2 tablespoon cilantros, chopped
- ☐ ¼ cup feta cheese, crumbled

## INSTRUCTIONS:

**1.** Add hummus to a serving dish. Add paprika and olive oil. Add olives, red bell pepper, feta cheese, pine nuts and cilantro, then mix well. Serve.

**PER SERVING:** Calories: 70 Carbs: 4g Fat: 5g Protein: 2g

# Smoky Loaded Eggplant Dip

**Preparation time:** 15 minutes

**Cooking time:** 20 minutes

**Servings:** 6

## INGREDIENTS:

- [ ] 1 large eggplant
- [ ] 1 ½ tablespoon Greek yoghurt
- [ ] 2 tablespoon tahini paste
- [ ] 1 garlic clove, chopped
- [ ] 1 tablespoon lemon juice
- [ ] 1 ½ teaspoon sumac
- [ ] ¾ teaspoon Aleppo pepper
- [ ] toasted pine nuts
- [ ] salt and pepper
- [ ] 1 tomato, diced
- [ ] ½ English cucumber, diced
- [ ] lemon juice
- [ ] parsley
- [ ] olive oil

## INSTRUCTIONS:

**1.** Add parsley, cucumber and tomato to a bowl. Season with ½

teaspoon sumac, salt and pepper. Add lemon juice and olive oil.

Toss and set aside.

**2.** Turn a gas burner on high and turn eggplant on it every 5 minutes with a tong until charred and crispy, for 20 minutes. Remove from the heat and let cool.

**3.** Peel the skin off the eggplant and discard the stem. Transfer eggplant flesh to a colander and drain for 5 minutes.

**4.** Transfer flesh to a blender. Add yoghurt, tahini paste, garlic, lemon juice, salt, pepper, Aleppo pepper and sumac. Blend for 2 pulses to combine.

**5.** Transfer to a bowl. Cover and refrigerate for 30 minutes. Bring it to a room temperature and add olive oil on top. Add pine nuts. Add salad on top and serve.

**PER SERVING:** Calories: 40 Carbs: 3g Fat: 4g Protein: 0g

# Peanut Butter Banana Greek Yogurt Bowl

**Preparation time:** 15 minutes

**Cooking time:** 0 minutes

**Servings:** 4

## INGREDIENTS:

- ☐ 2 medium bananas, sliced
- ☐ 4 cups vanilla Greek yoghurt
- ☐ ¼ cup peanut butter
- ☐ 1 teaspoon nutmeg
- ☐ ¼ cup flax seed meal

## INSTRUCTIONS:

**1.** Divide the yoghurt equally among 4 bowls and add banana slices

to it. Add peanut butter to a bowl and microwave for 40 seconds.

**2.** Add 1 tablespoon peanut butter over each bowl. Add nutmeg and

flax seed meal to each bowl. Serve.

**PER SERVING:** Calories: 110 Carbs: 13g Fat: 0g Protein: 15g

# Roasted Chickpeas

**Preparation time:** 15 minutes

**Cooking time:** 30 minutes

**Servings:** 2

## INGREDIENTS:

- [ ] 2 tablespoons extra virgin olive oil
- [ ] 2 15 oz. cans chickpeas
- [ ] 2 teaspoon red wine vinegar
- [ ] 2 teaspoon lemon juice
- [ ] 1 teaspoon dried oregano
- [ ] ½ teaspoon garlic powder
- [ ] 1 teaspoon kosher salt
- [ ] ½ teaspoon black pepper, cracked

## INSTRUCTIONS:

**1.** Preheat the oven to 425F and line a baking sheet with parchment paper. Drain, rinse and dry chickpeas and put on a baking sheet.

**2.** Roast for 10 minutes, then remove from the oven. Turn chickpeas and roast for 10 minutes. Add the remaining ingredients to a bowl and mix well.

**3.** Add chickpeas to it and mix to coat well. Transfer coated chickpeas back to the oven and roast for 10 minutes. Cool completely. Serve.

**PER SERVING:** Calories: 191 Carbs: 27g Fat: 1g Protein: 9g

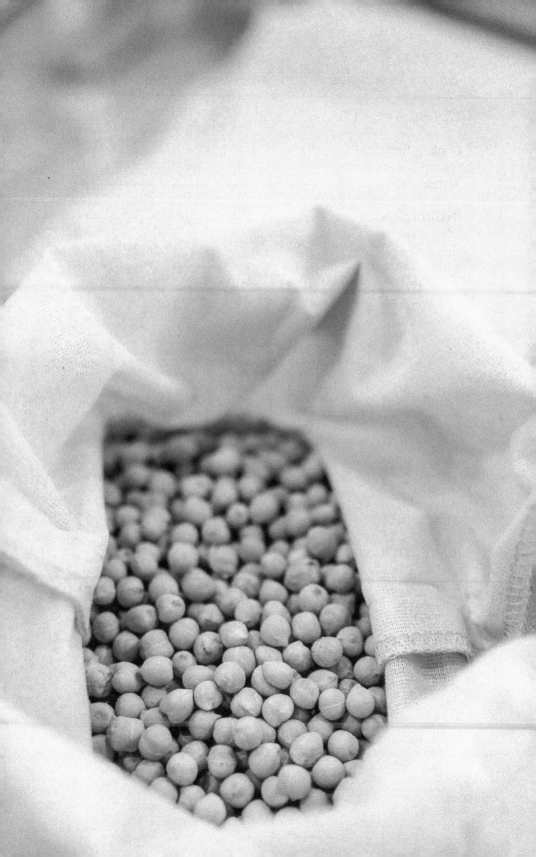

# Savory Feta Spinach and Sweet Red Pepper Muffins

**Preparation time:** 15 minutes

**Cooking time:** 25 minutes

**Servings:** 12

## INGREDIENTS:

- [ ] 2 eggs
- [ ] 2 ¾ cups all-purpose flour
- [ ] ¼ cup sugar
- [ ] 1 teaspoon paprika
- [ ] 2 teaspoons baking powder
- [ ] ¾ cup low-fat milk
- [ ] ½ cup extra virgin olive oil
- [ ] ¾ cup feta, crumbled
- [ ] 1/3 cup jarred florina peppers, drained and patted dry
- [ ] ¾ teaspoon salt
- [ ] 1 ¼ cup spinach, thinly sliced

## INSTRUCTIONS:

**1.** Preheat the oven to 375F. Mix sugar, flour, baking powder, paprika and salt in a bowl. Mix eggs, olive oil and milk in another bowl.

**2.** Add wet ingredients to dry and mix until blended. Add spinach, feta and peppers and mix well.

**3.** Line a muffin pan with liners and add the mixture to them equally. Bake for 25 minutes. Let cool for 10 minutes. Remove from the tray. Cool for 2 hours and serve.

**PER SERVING:** Calories: 295 Carbs: 27g Fat: 18g Protein: 8g

# Baked Whole-Grain Lavash Chips with Dip

**Preparation time:** 15 minutes

**Cooking time:** 6 minutes

**Servings:** 4

## INGREDIENTS:

- 3 teaspoon oil
- 3 California lavash whole-grain lavash flatbreads, cut into 16 squares
- 1 ripe avocado
- ½ cup cashews, soaked overnight, drained and rinsed
- ½ cup parsley, chopped
- 2 garlic cloves
- ½ cup kalamata olive brine
- ¼ cup tahini
- 1 lemon juice
- salt and pepper
- cherry tomatoes

## INSTRUCTIONS:

**1.** Blend cashews, avocado, garlic and parsley in a blender. Add lemon juice, olive brine, tahini and blend well. Season. Transfer to a bowl and add parsley. Set aside.

**2.** Preheat the oven to 400F and place lavash squares on top. Add little oil on both sides of each squares. Bake for 6 minutes and remove from the oven Let cool.

**3.** Chop cherry tomatoes. Serve chips with tomatoes and dip.

**PER SERVING:** Calories: 557 Carbs: 33g Fat: 30g Protein: 35g

# Quinoa Granola

**Preparation time:** 15 minutes

**Cooking time:** 35 minutes

**Servings:** 7

## INGREDIENTS:

- ☐ 1 cup old fashioned rolled oats
- ☐ 2 cups raw almonds, chopped
- ☐ ½ cup white quinoa, uncooked
- ☐ 1 tablespoon coconut sugar
- ☐ 3 ½ tablespoon coconut oil
- ☐ ¼ cup maple syrup
- ☐ pinch sea salt

## INSTRUCTIONS:

**1.** Preheat the oven to 340F. Add quinoa, oats, almonds, sugar and salt to a bowl. Mix well. Add maple syrup and coconut oil to a pan. Heat over medium heat for 3 minutes, whisking along.

**2.** Add dry ingredients and stir to coat well. Place on a baking sheet and spread. Bake for 20 minutes. Remove from the oven and toss the granola.

**3.** Turn pan around and bake for 8 minutes more. Cool completely and serve.

**PER SERVING:** Calories: 274 Carbs: 38g Fat: 11g Protein: 9g

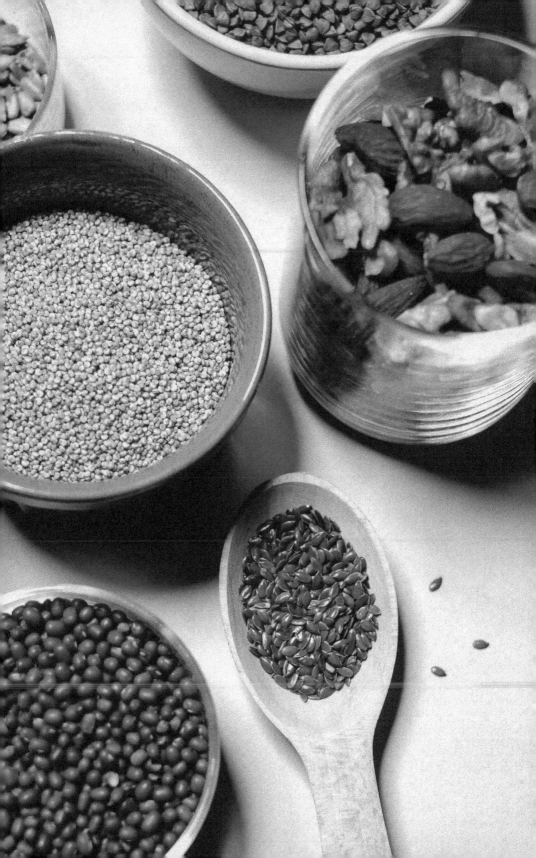

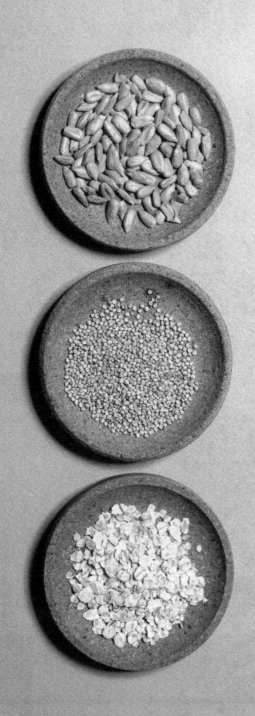

CPSIA information can be obtained
at www.ICGtesting.com
Printed in the USA
LVHW081713270521
688665LV00015B/883

9 781802 328479